EYE CARE
EYE WEAR

for Better Vision

by Mark Rossi

Amberwood Publishing Ltd
Park Corner, Park Horsley, East Horsley, Surrey KT24 5RZ
Telephone: 01483 285919

ISBN 1-899308-01-6

Cover design by Design Hive

Typeset and designed by
Word Perfect, Christchurch, Dorset.

Printed in Great Britain

CONTENTS

Note to Reader

Foreword

All Optometrists have to obtain a university degree in Optometry followed by twelve months in practice with a suitably qualified supervisor. During this time further examinations have to be passed. These consist of practical and oral sessions set by the British College of Optometrists covering all aspects of the practice of Optometry. Every section has to be passed before students can be registered with the General Optical Council. Only then are they allowed to take the responsibility of conducting eye examinations on the public.

All through the learning process a vast amount of knowledge and skill is assimilated and can be used to the advantage of the patient. It would be completely impossible to convey the principles of Optometry in any comprehensive fashion in a short publication, therefore any attempt will be an individual interpretation of the essentials in the light of experience.

This book is just such an interpretation which sets out to summarise the knowledge and range of skills which are used to conduct an eye examination, to investigate the health of the various parts of the eye, and to give advice regarding the use of the eyes under all circumstances. This is done in terms which can be understood by anyone, and in such a way that a complete overall picture is portrayed. It will help greatly in making the right choice of Optometrist and in understanding what to expect in a properly conducted comprehensive eye examination by a caring professional.

I believe that a more informed public is a desirable thing. It should lead to a more discriminating patient, and in the long run to a more efficient and better Optometric Service. This indeed is the sole purpose of this book.

C I McPherson FBCO
President
British College of Optometrists 1994/95

*This book is proudly dedicated to all those fine people
who helped me in its preparation,
they know who they are.*

1 | Introduction

The purpose of this book is to demystify opticians and provide an insight to eye care and eye wear. It presents practical information and an understanding of optical considerations, enabling the consumer to make informed decisions.

Mankind is primarily visually-motivated as sight accounts for eighty percent of the five senses combined. The loss of visual function is devastating, yet more time and money is spent on hair care than on eye care! Eye protection should be a major consideration for everyone, yet eyes go unguarded too often.

The eye is a unique organ in the body, as its intricate interior may be minutely examined non-invasively through the pupil, the window to the inside of the eye. Changes observed in the transparent, small arteries and veins in the retina at the back of the eye, give an indication of the state of blood vessels throughout the body. This enables the detection of many general diseases which manifest themselves in the eye, such as high blood pressure, narrowing of arteries by fatty deposits and diabetes. The eye is diagnostically the most useful cubic inch of your body.

The structures that make up the eye are described with their function, associated disorders and typical treatments. This will serve as a useful guide in the recognition of the common eye disorders.

Lenses were in use before the time of Christ and have helped to shape human history through such inventions as spectacles, the microscope, the telescope and the camera. Fittingly, technology now offers a bewildering choice of lens materials and designs to overcome specific drawbacks without sacrificing optical integrity.

The purpose of the procedures performed in the eye examination are revealed. The nature of sight defects and their related symptoms are explained in detail, and the myths surrounding the consequences of bad habits are dispelled. It will then become apparent that the cause of a sight defect is not an unhealthy eye, but rather one requiring correction. This knowledge permits objective criticism concerning 'cures' for sight defects to be made.

In recent years eye surgery has become available for the correction of sight defects. However, it would be unwise to have irreversible eye surgery whilst harbouring false expectations. Advances in contact lens materials and designs have made this type of correction first choice for many. By comparing the alternatives to spectacles a judgement of their suitability can be made.

Visual Display Units (VDUs) are in everyday use by many people, at work and at home, and have been associated with a wide variety of problems. The ergonomic adjustments which can improve visual and physical comfort are explored, together with the guidelines from the Health and Safety Executive governing those working with display screen equipment.

2 | Visiting the Optician

The receptionist is responsible for booking appointments for an eye examination. Previous eye examinations carried out at that practice should be mentioned together with details of whether contact lenses are worn or desired. A home visit can be requested, but it is only appropriate in compelling circumstances. It is better to be examined at the practice, where all the necessary equipment is readily available.

Since 1st April 1989, there has been a private fee for an eye examination. However, about 40% of the populace qualify for a 'free' National Health Service (NHS) eye examination by being in one of the following categories:

- Low income;
- Income Support or Family Credit;
- Under 16 or a full-time student under 19;
- Very strong lenses;
- Registered blind or partially sighted;
- Diabetic or glaucoma sufferer;
- Over 40 and the parent, brother, sister or child of glaucoma sufferer;
- Hospital Eye Service patient.

The upper four groups are also entitled to a NHS Voucher to help towards the cost of spectacles or contact lenses.

Compared with our ancestors, modern man makes many demands on his visual system in the course of everyday living. Often such demands result from conditions where the eyes are subjected to prolonged stress, often involuntary and unsuspected, where some degree of eyestrain is inevitable. Every year approximately one quarter of the UK population have their eyes examined; over 90% are performed by registered optometrists (ophthalmic opticians), the remainder are conducted by ophthalmic medical practitioners. Their role is not merely to give clear vision, but to relieve discomfort and to achieve maximum efficiency at various tasks.

An eye examination covers the following areas:

- Detection of any abnormality of the eye, for example glaucoma, at an early stage when improvement, containment or cure can be achieved with proper treatment;
- Professional evaluation of the standard of vision, focusing ability, eye co-ordination, field of vision, colour vision and depth perception;
- Accurate determination of the prescription, this is the exact specification of lenses needed to optimise vision;
- Informed advice to achieve all visual requirements, including safety spectacles, VDU and driving standards. (Remember even qualified drivers are legally required to be able to read a normal car number plate from a distance of seventy-five feet in good daylight with spectacles or contact lenses if normally worn);
- Prescribing spectacles, contact lenses or low visual aid.

The patient should receive a copy of the prescription by right, which is valid for two years, and be advised of any change or if referral to a GP is indicated. A personal record card must be kept for a minimum of eight years and patients have access to entries made after November 1991.

The **ophthalmic medical practitioner** (OMP) is a qualified doctor who specialises in eyes and will check the health of the eyes and determine the prescription. There are about eight hundred registered with the General Optical Council (GOC) in the UK.

The **optometrist** is a graduate professional – a requirement since the Opticians Act 1958 – who will check the health of the eyes, determine the prescription, advise on visual problems, and who may supply and fit spectacles or contact lenses. There are over six thousand registered with the GOC in the UK, and many also belong to other professional organisations.

The specialities are:

- Contact lenses by gaining the Diploma in Contact Lens Practice (DCLP);
- Orthoptic therapy to develop or restore the ability of both eyes to work together binocularly;
- Low visual aids, microscopic and telescopic optical appliances to improve the vision of the partially sighted;
- Occupational optometry, which is concerned with lighting and visual efficiency at work, VDU equipment and eye protection;
- Paediatric or children's visual problems. (Parents should bring their children for an eye examination at about three years of age, or sooner,

if an eye problem is suspected or there is a history of poor vision in the family. Most eye diseases found in the very young can be successfully treated if detected at an early stage);

• Sports vision, to improve performance by specific visual training.

Increasingly it will be the **dispensing optician** who advises on which spectacles are most suited to individual lifestyle, vocation, sporting and leisure needs, and makes the accurate measurements necessary to supply and fit them. There are over three thousand registered with the GOC in the UK, and some specially certified may fit contact lenses to a prescription.

Since December 1984 **unregistered** personnel with no optical qualifications may dispense spectacles to a prescription not more than two years old, but not to children under the age of sixteen years, or patients registered blind or partially sighted.

Spectacles or contact lenses do not have to be purchased from the practice where the eyes were examined. Since 1989, opticians have been able to advertise both their services and promotions. However, the dispensing of certain lens types requires an adjustment to the prescription, obliging the supplier to contact the prescriber for approval. A practice offering a 'free' or heavily discounted fee for an eye examination hopes for an increased revenue from the supply of spectacles or contact lenses to subsidise those not dispensed.

A registered practice will supply suitable, durable spectacles, to British Standards specifications, and position the optical centres of both lenses accurately in the frame to correspond exactly with the eyes' separation. The Health and Medicines Act 1988 allows for the purchase, from non-optical outlets, of ready-made reading spectacles, which assume that both eyes require the same power and are averagely separated. Their use should be confined to occasional brief close work or where there is a high risk of soiling, for example decorating, and do not replace a regular eye examination.

The quality of frames is not always related to their price. Beware of discontinued frames, if they are broken a replacement cannot easily be ordered from the manufacturer. Make enquiries as to whether the spectacles are guaranteed, the duration of cover, it should be at least one year, and any exception clauses that would invalidate a future claim. When collecting spectacles check vision and examine them closely for the presence of uneven tints, rough edges, insecure hinges, and gaps between the lens and frame. The lenses should be as close to the eyes as possible without touching the eyelashes. When the spectacles are securely installed they should fit snugly behind the ears, and not slip down to rest on the cheeks. To maintain optimum comfort return regularly to have the spectacles re-adjusted.

For best results visually and aesthetically, spectacles should be washed regularly in warm, soapy water to keep them clean and sparkling. Do not clean lenses with paper tissues, a dirty cloth or a tie, as they can scratch. If spectacles are hung on a cord around the neck, take care not to scratch the lenses. Spectacles should be removed by grasping them with both hands close to the hinges, an habitual one-handed dismount causes the frame to bend or break. The best place to store spectacles is in a case; a hard case is better than a soft one.

The appropriate time interval between eye examinations depends on many factors, most people receive a reminder card after about two years. Continuity enables a useful history to be established, which may prove important in charting minor changes enabling the early diagnosis of other medical conditions. However, if you are not completely satisfied with previous treatment, then select another practice using the following criteria:

- Is recommended by friends or GP;
- Allows at least twenty minutes for the consultation;
- The dust covers have been removed from modern instruments;
- Has a good selection of suitable spectacles;
- Displays names and qualifications of practitioners.

What further action can be taken if a complaint to an optician has not been satisfactorily resolved?

Those examined under the NHS should approach the local Family Health Services Authority within thirteen weeks of the consultation, their address will be available in the practice or the local library.

Disputes concerning services, spectacles or contact lenses, which cannot be resolved at branch or head-office level, are dealt with by the Optical Consumer Complaints Service (OCCS), their address is given in chapter 11.

Cases of professional misconduct should be directed to the General Optical Council (GOC), the governing body of the optical professions, their address is given in chapter 11.

3 | Common eye disorders

If an injury, disease or abnormality is suspected a referral letter, detailing the findings with a provisional diagnosis, will be sent to the general practitioner (GP) concerned or, in an urgent case, directly to casualty. GPs may treat; styes, bacterial conjunctivitis, superficial trauma to the lids, cornea and conjunctiva, and superficial corneal foreign bodies. The more serious eye diseases or symptoms will be referred to an ophthalmologist, a medical doctor who specialises in the diagnosis, treatment and surgery of the eyes.

3.1 ANATOMY OF THE EYE WITH ASSOCIATED DISORDERS
Each part of the eye is specialised to perform a specific function.

Below is a section through the eye.

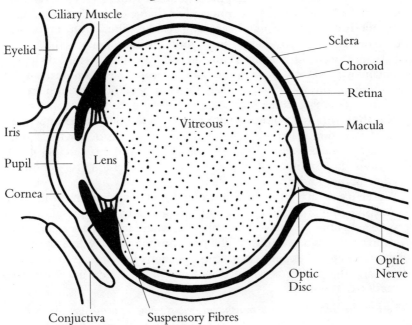

The eyelids are movable, protective folds of muscle fibres, covered by thin skin on the outside and lined by a thin layer of conjunctiva on the inner surface. The eyelashes grow from the lid margins; there are also two openings to allow the drainage of tears, and the tiny outlets of the oil-secreting and sweat-secreting glands. Blinking spreads a thin layer of salty tears evenly over the cornea, on average fifteen times a minute, to keep the eye clean and moist.

Blepharitis is a very common chronic relapsing inflammation of the eyelid margins which are red and scaly and, in severe cases, swollen and ulcerated. It begins early in childhood and frequently continues throughout life. The most important factor in its treatment is cleanliness, which is best maintained by rubbing the scales from the eyelid margins daily, either with a hot, wet clean cotton bud or by scrubbing using a baby shampoo. The disorder is associated with bacterial infection and, frequently, dandruff so a vigorous attempt should be made to keep the scalp clean.

Stye is a red painful swelling of pus, usually caused by bacterial infection of a sweat-secreting gland of an eyelash follicle. It is similar to a boil elsewhere on the skin. Styes tend to occur in groups, because the bacteria spread from one hair follicle to another, either directly or by the fingers. Antibiotic ointment may prevent further infection. Heat can give mild relief and encourages pointing and discharge of the abscess.

Chalazion is a cyst of an oil-secreting gland resulting from a blockage of the outlet, characterised by a hard, round painless lump in the eyelid. Chalazions occur in persons of any age and about one third disappear spontaneously. With increase in size it may cause astigmatism by distortion of the eye. It is excised through a vertical incision of the conjunctival surface under local anaesthetic.

Xanthelasma is a yellowish fatty deposit in the skin of the upper and lower lids, common in the elderly. It merits an investigation in the young, since it represents a raised level of cholesterol or other fats in the blood. It causes no symptoms but may require excision for cosmetic considerations, under local anaesthetic.

Watering, with tears overflowing onto the cheek occurring principally in one eye only, may be caused by a foreign body or, if present over a prolonged period, by an obstruction somewhere in the passage draining tears from the two openings in the eyelid to the nose. When the social embarrassment of regurgitated tears, possibly infected, is sufficiently distressing the passage is syringed with warm salt water, but if this fails surgery is necessary.

The conjunctiva is the thin translucent, moist, mucus membrane covering the front white part of the eye and the inside of the eyelids. It has a rich supply of blood vessels, normally nearly invisible, and is very sensitive.

Hyperaemia is an excessive amount of blood in the dilated conjunctival vessels caused by fatigue, excessive reading, poor ventilation, excessive dryness or exposure to smog, smoke, dust, wind, air pollutants, strong light and heat. The redness and soreness may be relieved by the use of artificial tear drops, cold compresses or drugs to narrow the blood vessels.

Conjunctivitis is very common, usually affecting both eyes causing redness, swelling and watering, accompanied by a sensation of burning or grittiness. To limit transfer of infection, individual clean face-cloths and towels should be used. It may be caused by the following:

Allergy to pollen (hay fever), mascara, chlorine in swimming pools, or preservatives used in eye-drops and contact lens solutions.

Bacterial conjunctivitis with a sticky discharge of mucus and pus, which causes the eyelids to be stuck together on awakening, responds to broad-spectrum antibiotic drops within three days.

Chlamydial conjunctivitis known as trachoma, prevalent in underdeveloped tropical countries, if not treated with tetracycline ointment, can lead to blindness by extensively scarring the cornea.

Viral conjunctivitis with profuse watery discharge, for which there is no specific treatment, is highly contagious and lasts up to three weeks.

Pinguecula is a harmless small, oval, yellowish-white spot on the conjunctiva, usually on the nasal side. It is very common after middle age but requires no treatment.

Pterygium is a triangular fold of vascularized conjunctival membrane that extends onto the cornea from the nasal conjunctiva. Common in tropical climates where an outdoor existence exposes the eyes to harmful ultraviolet sunlight, wind and dust. Surgical excision stunts its growth and counters visual impairment, although the incidence of recurrence is high.

Subconjunctival haemorrhage is the sudden appearance of an irregular red patch under the conjunctiva, caused by the spreading of blood from a ruptured conjunctival blood vessel. It may occur spontaneously or following concerted coughing, straining, lifting or vigorous sneezing, usually no treatment is required, the blood is absorbed in about two weeks, changing colour from bright red to yellow. However, repeated attacks may be indicative of blood disorders, high blood pressure or diabetes.

The cornea is the circular, transparent, tough coating of the eye over the iris and pupil. The thickness varies from 1mm in the periphery to 0.5mm in the centre.

However, during sleep, it swells by about 4%. Since it has no blood supply, it cannot fend off infection easily. On insult, the outer layer heals rapidly by regeneration, and because it has numerous nerve fibres, it is extremely sensitive.

Corneal abrasions are superficial scratches and erosions of the cornea, which cause watering and severe pain, especially with movement of the lid over the cornea. They may be seen as disturbed reflections from a torch, while fluorescent dye will stain the abrasions green. Rarely, imperfect healing leads to a recurrence, typically several weeks or months later when opening the eye upon awakening, which usually heals within a few hours.

Arcus senilis is the gradual deposition of a grey-white ring of fat in the peripheral cornea of both eyes, seen in most elderly people. In the young it may be indicative of abnormally high fat levels in the blood.

The iris is a ring of muscles giving the eye its colour (blue, brown, grey, green or hazel), and by contracting or dilating is able to shrink or enlarge the size of the pupil.

Iritis is inflammation of the iris, usually confined to one eye, with blurring of vision and intense light sensitivity. The eye becomes painful from spasm of the iris and ciliary muscles. There is also reddening surrounding the cornea. Eye-drops to relieve the pain by paralysing the iris and ciliary muscles cause the pupil to widen and prevent reading. Vigorous treatment by steroids to suppress the inflammation is usually effective within ten days. However, recurrences commonly occur in either eye.

The lens is optically clear having no blood or nerve supply. The firm centre is surrounded by softer, concentric layers of fibres, contained in an elastic, fibrous capsule. The lens is suspended by numerous fine fibres attached to the ciliary muscle, which by contracting or relaxing allows the lens to alter shape for focusing nearby objects.

Cataract is present when the lens becomes progressively opaque, causing the pupil to appear a cloudy grey or white instead of black, giving misty distance vision but clearer near vision initially. It is an irreversible sign of ageing, the protein of the lens becomes denatured, as in a hard-boiled egg or the whitening of the hair. It may also be caused by injury, steroid drugs, diabetes and infrared radiation. Dazzle caused by the scattering of light is pronounced in bright sunlight, this is alleviated by wearing a wide brimmed hat. Night driving is affected by oncoming headlights having coloured rings or haloes around them. When the decreasing vision in the better eye prevents the sufferer from leading a normal life, the lens in the poorer eye needs to be extracted surgically. In the majority of elderly patients a plastic replacement intraocular lens implant is inserted into the eye calculated to provide best vision, although reading spectacles will be necessary.

Dislocated lens is usually caused by an injury that ruptures the supporting fibres, this severely impairs vision and may also cause glaucoma necessitating lens removal.

The vitreous is a transparent jelly, consisting almost entirely of water, filling the large cavity between the lens and retina, giving the eye its shape, with ageing the gel breaks down in part becoming liquid.

Floaters are aggregations of very tiny fragments floating in the vitreous which cast a shadow on the retina, being seen as fine, dark spots darting about in the field of vision on eye movement, but only drifting slightly when the eyes are still. They vary in size and shape, being especially visible when reading or looking at a plain, light background, often imaginatively described as flies, spiders or worms. They are very common in the short-sighted and middle aged, but require no treatment as with time they descend under gravity out of the line of sight.

In more than half of the over 60s, especially the short-sighted, the vitreous may normally spontaneously collapse and detach from the retina. This may be accompanied by the **sudden** onset of **many** floaters and 'flashing lights' where the vitreous continues to pull on the retina, which in about 5% of cases will result in a retinal tear. A retinal tear may be sealed either by laser or by the application of extreme cold. Left untreated there is a high risk of a retinal detachment.

The retina is a thin layer of light-sensitive nerve cells, called rods and cones, lining the inside of the eye, which convert light into electrical impulses which are transmitted to the brain along the optic nerve.

Retinal detachment may follow major injury to the eye or, more usually, occur spontaneously, presenting as a sudden loss of vision, a shower of floaters, 'flashing lights' or an increasing shadow in the field of vision. Hospitalisation to rejoin the detached retina to the underlying choroid by the application of extreme cold, is often effective if undertaken soon after the onset.

3.2 GLAUCOMA

In **glaucoma** part or all of the vision is lost by excessive pressure within the eye, acting on the optic disc, causing irreversible damage to the optic nerve either directly or indirectly by interfering with the blood supply.

In **chronic** glaucoma the pressure in the eye, usually both, rises gradually over a period of years, causing a slow, progressive, painless loss of peripheral vision. It is usually unnoticed in the early stages, but if untreated irretrievably extinguishes all vision. It rarely occurs before the age of 40 years, after which it affects about one in two hundred of the general population. There is a high risk of glaucoma in those who have a family history, diabetes, high short-sightedness or of Afro-Caribbean origin. There is no cure; it is controlled by daily eye-drops that reduce the eye pressure to prevent further visual field loss. Both the eye pressure and visual fields must be measured periodically throughout life.

In **acute** glaucoma dilation of the pupil causes the pressure in the eye to rise rapidly to high levels over a few hours, with a marked decrease in vision, severe pain and occasionally nausea. The affected eye appears red, the cornea becomes misty and the pupil is semi-dilated, oval and fixed. It usually affects the long-sighted over the age of 40 years, occurring in about one in a thousand of the general population. Surgical treatment within hours to reduce the pressure is needed to prevent a substantial and permanent loss of vision. There may be a history of previous subacute attacks lasting a few hours, especially at night, where vision becomes blurred, the eye aches and lights appear to have coloured rainbow haloes.

3.3 SQUINT OR EYETURN

Squint, known technically as strabismus, occurs when both eyes cannot simultaneously be directed at the same object. Each eye is rotated easily by six muscles attached to the outer surface and may be compared to reins on a team of horses. The deviating eye may turn **in** 'cross-eyed', **out** 'wall-eyed' or, less commonly, **up** or **down**. Since the two eyes do not co-ordinate, their separate images are too markedly different to be fused to achieve true depth perception; important when judging distance.

In a **paralytic** squint, which generally affects adults, one or more of the six eye muscles are paralysed. The characteristic deviation between the two eyes is sudden and variable, causing the distressing sensation of double vision, which sufferers may reduce by an altered head posture. Double vision occurring in any person over five years old requires investigation by a neurologist within a day. It may indicate a brain tumour, stroke, disease of the nerves supplying the eye muscles such as multiple sclerosis, disease of the eye muscles themselves as in Graves' disease, fracture of the bony eye socket, diabetes, high blood pressure or hyperthyroidism.

In **non-paralytic** squint there is no eye muscle weakness, so the amount of deviation between the two eyes is constant. It is very common, often being hereditary, occurring either within a few weeks of birth or between the ages of about three and four years. The brain adapts to avoid the troublesome double vision by suppressing the vision of the deviating eye. It is caused most commonly by excessive long-sightedness or from sensory deprivation in one eye preventing fixation, for example cataract. When spectacles and eye exercises, to develop binocular vision, fail to correct the squint, surgical intervention is necessary to align the eyes. Treatment by patching the good eye, to improve the undeveloped vision in the previously deviating eye, is not usually successful after the age of eight years; this permanently reduced vision is known as amblyopia.

4 | Lenses

In the year 1268, Roger Bacon an English Franciscan monk advocated the use of lenses to aid persons of weak sight; this effectively lengthened their useful lives.

4.1 LENS OPTICS

Sunlight travelling in a straight line at 186,000 miles per second takes eight minutes to reach the Earth. Visualise holding a magnifying glass and focusing sunlight onto a piece of paper. The parallel light rays from the sun are bent by the magnifying glass causing them to *converge*. By adjusting the distance between the magnifying glass and the paper the sunlight may be brought into sharp focus. This distance is known as the focal length of the lens, a concept introduced by the German mathematician Gauss.

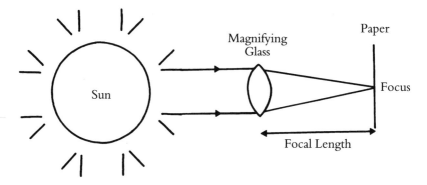

The focal length of a convex lens

If you measure the focal length with a metric ruler, then the reciprocal or inverse expresses the power of the magnifying glass in dioptres, the shorter the focal length of a lens, the greater the lens power. For example, the power of a lens of two metre focal length is half a dioptre, a one metre focal length is one dioptre and a half a metre focal length is two dioptres.

When a magnifying glass is used, the object to be examined is placed at the focal distance of the lens, to produce a magnified image. A four dioptre magnifying glass enables perusal at one quarter of a metre.

The Chinese introduced the prototype ready-made reading spectacles in the tenth century by glazing magnifying glasses into frames. A magnifying glass is a convex lens, being thicker at the centre than at the edge.

A concave lens is thicker at the edge than at the centre and diminishes the size of an object seen through it. A concave lens will bend light rays from a distant object making them spread apart so that they never meet. If the lines along which they *diverge* are traced backwards towards the incoming light, although there are no actual rays present they appear to meet at an imaginary focus, shown on the diagram below to the left of the lens.

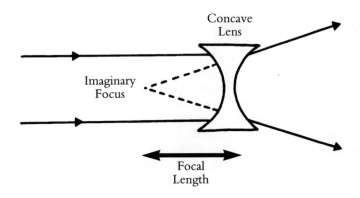

The focal length of a concave lens

Both the above lenses may be thought of as sections of a spherical surface and are therefore known as spherical lenses. All the light rays that pass through a spherical lens come to a focal **point**.

A class of lenses which may be considered as sections of a cylindrical surface are known as cylindrical lenses. They have one plane surface with no power, along which light rays pass undeviated, and at right angles, a curved surface with maximum power, along which light rays are bent to a focal *line*.

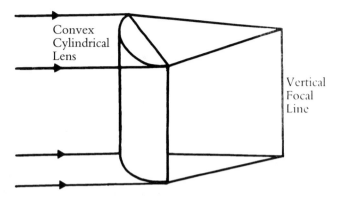

Convex
Cylindrical
Lens

Vertical
Focal
Line

The focal length of a convex cylindrical lens

4.2 LENS MATERIALS

The earliest spectacle lenses were emerald, amethyst, topaz and ruby. When these were deemed as ostentatious, quartz (pebble lenses) was substituted. Quartz has now fallen from favour as it is expensive. Spectacle lenses today are made from either a high-quality glass or, more usually, plastic. They must be free of flaws, bubbles and surface irregularities, and are designed to minimise aberrations which impair the quality of the image by loss of definition (blurring), distortion (wrong shape) and chromatism (colour fringes).

There are many types of **glass** used for spectacle lenses. **Crown** glass is the most common; **photochromic** glass reacts automatically to changing light conditions, darkening in sunlight and lightening indoors; **ultraviolet-absorbing** glass shields the eye from harmful radiation; and **high-index** glass produces a thinner high-power lens. A heat or chemically treated 'toughened' glass lens offers eye protection by being impact-resistant and crumbling into 'hailstones' rather than sharp splinters, when broken.

There are many types of **plastics** used for spectacle lenses. The original perspex (**PMMA**); allyl diglycol carbonate introduced in the late 1950's as Columbia Resin (**CR-39**); **high-index** plastic for a thinner, lighter high-power lens; and **polycarbonate** for a high impact-resistant lens. Plastic lenses are only half the weight of glass lenses, but are appreciably thicker and scratch more easily. It is advisable to have an invisible scratch-resistant quartz hard coating on the front surface where ninety percent of scratches occur. On the rare occasion when a plastic lens does fracture, it breaks into large blunt-edged pieces, and is therefore recommended for children and active adults.

A laminated lens has a thin layer of plastic sandwiched between two pieces of glass. If the lens is shattered, the glass fragments adhere to the unbroken plastic sheet, reducing the risk of injury to the face and eyes.

4.3 LENS COATINGS

Not all the light striking a lens passes through, some eight percent is reflected back by the front and back surfaces, more so for high-index lenses. An **anti-reflection** (**AR**) coating on both surfaces of the lens significantly increases the total light transmission, reducing ghost images, which are especially noticeable to very short-sighted people with thick lenses. It also makes the lens look thinner to other people and gives them a clearer view of the eye. There are three types of AR coatings; single layer, multi-layer and broadband. Their properties and appearance can vary with the lens material to which they are applied. Careful cleaning and avoidance of hair-spray is necessary to preserve the AR coating for several years.

A **tint** selectively absorbs light of its observable colour or bands in the invisible spectrum, for example ultraviolet or infrared which are harmful to the eye. A plastic lens may have an even or graduated tint of any colour or shade chemically coated over the outside surface, being removable if desired. A glass lens formerly had the tint throughout, so the thicker the lens, the darker and more uneven the colour; nowadays the tint is more often vacuum coated. Choose sunglasses that conform to British Standard BS 2724:1987 to be sure of adequate eye protection.

A neutral grey tint reduces the light intensity across the visible spectrum equally, without the loss of colour differentiation and is useful for light sensitive people. A green tint reduces ultraviolet and infrared light, making violet, blue, orange or red colours less distinguishable. A brown tint will eliminate almost all of the ultraviolet and imbues a sense of 'warmness'. A blue tint assists the judgement of the temperature in a blast furnace, but offers little eye protection. A yellow tint reduces ultraviolet, violet and blue, thereby enhancing the contrast of red and green, but making shadows darker still. Other colour tints are mainly cosmetic. In marginal light conditions, for example dawn, dusk and fog, tinted lenses reduce visibility and should not be worn for driving. In all cases too dark a tint will dilate the pupil giving less distinct vision and can exaggerate shadows and lines around the eyes.

A **polarised** lens reduces horizontally reflected glare from flat 'shiny' surfaces, such as glass and water, allowing true colour appreciation.

4.4 LENS FORMS

Spectacle lenses have both front and back surfaces curved in the same direction but by different amounts, as this produces a better image, is cosmetically more attractive and allows the scanning eye to remain close to the lens.

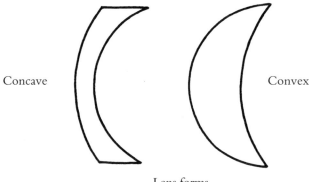

Concave   Convex

Lens forms

A **single vision** lens has the same power over its entire surface. It may be used for both distance and near vision until middle age, when separate reading spectacles are required. Some opticians stock single vision lenses and may produce complete spectacles to a prescription in hours.

The switching between distance and reading spectacles was sufficiently inconvenient to the American statesman Benjamin Franklin in the eighteenth century that he wore spectacles with the two separate lenses cut in half and joined together. A **bifocal** lens has a telltale dividing line separating the top portion used for distance vision from the lower

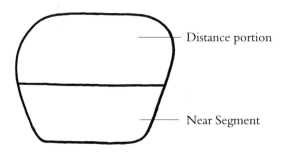

— Distance portion

— Near Segment

'Executive' bifocal

segment used for near vision. The knack to effective use is to lower the eyes to read rather than tilting the head, although it takes a while to become accustomed. Bifocals are particularly useful when, for example, one is writing notes from a blackboard.

There are many types of bifocal lenses to suit a wide variety of purposes. The larger and more conspicuous the near segment, the wider the field of view, but then negotiating stairs can become hazardous, unless the head is tilted to look down to foot level through the distance portion.

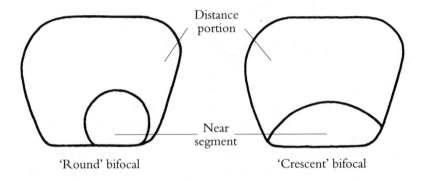

'Round' bifocal   'Crescent' bifocal

As the eye rotates down to read it crosses the dividing line which causes near objects to apparently 'jump' upward, like a jack-in-the-box. This disturbance may be minimised by having a near segment with as straight a top as possible, which also gives a greater useful area for close work.

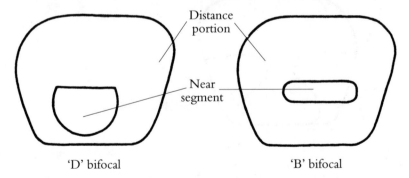

'D' bifocal   'B' bifocal

With advancing years detailed objects just beyond the range of near vision are seen indistinctly. A **trifocal** lens has a small *specific* intermediate area to overcome this problem, situated between the distance and near vision areas, which may be tricky to adapt to initially.

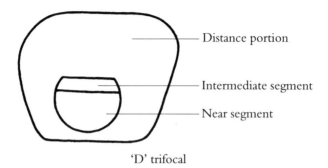

Distance portion

Intermediate segment

Near segment

'D' trifocal

Introduced in 1959 the **varifocal** or **progressive** lens has a gradual increase in power along an invisible corridor, bridging the top and bottom zones of the lens, and looks like a single vision lens.

The narrow reading area compared to bifocals, necessitates more lateral head movement when reading and a frame shape which does not restrict the lower nasal area. The corridor permits distinct vision at *any* intermediate position, without objects apparently 'jumping', by the technique of pointing the nose at what is to be viewed and raising the chin to achieve maximum clarity.

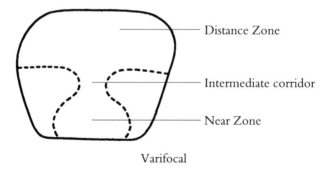

Distance Zone

Intermediate corridor

Near Zone

Varifocal

The distorted vision either side of the corridor causes a disturbing 'rocking' sensation on horizontal eye movement, until learned to be ignored after two to four weeks wear. To lessen this effect, a soft design progressive lens was launched in 1973 with a wider corridor – being more suited to sustained intermediate vision, such as VDU work – but having a slightly blurred peripheral distance vision and an even narrower reading area. However, for regular intermediate use, trifocals are more efficient.

Varifocals must be very precisely fitted in the frame and are available in many varieties to satisfy different needs.

5 | Sight defects

To appreciate the nature of optical sight defects, it is necessary to understand the underlying optical principles of lenses, described in section 4.1, and to have some familiarity with the optics of the normal eye.

5.1 OPTICS OF THE NORMAL EYE

Leonardo da Vinci in the fifteenth century imagined the futuristic photographic camera to be analogous optically with the eye, with the pupil acting as a variable aperture, a lens system and a retina that corresponds to the film.

The sense of sight depends upon light rays from an object changing direction as they pass through the cornea and lens to focus on the retina, the total optical power being equivalent to a magnifying glass with a magnification of fifteen. The image is inverted and reversed with respect to the object. However, the mind perceives objects in the upright position despite the upside down orientation on the retina because the brain is trained to consider an inverted image as the normal.

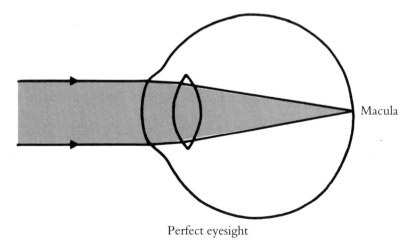

Macula

Perfect eyesight

In perfect eyesight, the image of a distant object, anything farther than six metres away, is formed accurately on the most sensitive part of the retina known as the macula. The ciliary muscle of the eye is relaxed, so that the power of the lens is least. This condition is called **emmetropia** ('sight in proper measure').

Light rays from an object closer than six metres are divergent. Therefore to photograph a nearby object with a camera it is necessary to move the lens away from the film to focus for a clear picture. Since the lens in the eye cannot be moved, when we read a book the ciliary muscle must contract to allow the lens to become thicker, giving a more convex shape with greater converging power. This focusing or accommodation is achieved instantaneously without conscious thought, being a largely reflex mechanism, enabling the divergent light rays of close objects to be focused clearly on the macula.

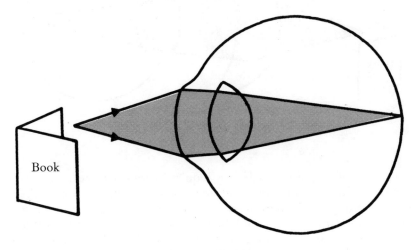

Focusing on a close object

That the eye has the power of accommodation is proved by attempting to look through the meshes of a net at a distant object, we cannot see both the meshes and the object with equal clarity at the same time. With ageing, the lens becomes progressively stiffer and less flexible, owing to irreversible chemical changes, such that the ciliary muscle, even trying maximally, is less able to adjust the lens' shape to focus for close vision.

This causes blurring of near vision, known as **presbyopia** ('old sight') and by the age of sixty the lens is unable to change shape at all. The decline is most striking between the age of thirty years, when a book may be read at twelve centimetres, and forty years, when a book cannot be read closer than twenty-two centimetres.

When a newspaper has to be held at arm's length to see it clearly, or an individual has difficulty reading fine print, aggravated in dim illumination, possibly associated with frontal headache and visual fatigue, reading spectacles are necessary. The average person first requires reading spectacles between the ages of forty-two and forty-five years.

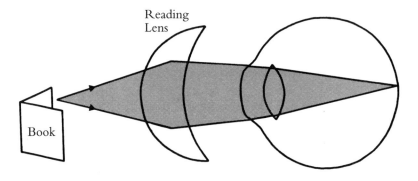

Convex lens assisting focusing

The power of the spectacle lens required varies with an individual's habits, age, occupation and accustomed distance of doing near work. A new prescription is required about every two years to make up for the loss of accommodative power, until the late fifties, at which time the reading spectacles accomplish most of the change in focus required for close work. Reading spectacles will blur distant objects and should not be worn when walking. They do not contribute to the further loss of accommodation or affect the health of the eye, for better or worse.

5.2 SIGHT DEFECTS

Most people have a sight defect, whereby the image of a distant object focuses either in front of or behind the macula. As this is generally dependent on the length of the eye the final outcome will not be evident until the eye stops growing in the early twenties. Sight defects, known technically as **ametropia** ('sight not in proper measure'), are largely hereditarily determined but in no definitely predictable way, since they are also influenced by the shape of the cornea and lens. Headache, dizziness and occasionally nausea may have their origin in a sight defect.

In addition to the visual disturbance caused by sight defects, a child may display blinking, frowning, rubbing the eyes, head tilting, closing one eye, crossed eyes, clumsiness, light sensitivity, redness of the eye and watering. This must be distinguished from the child who sits close to the television screen for the specific purpose of enjoying a larger, easier picture to view, with a greater sense of involvement with the story.

▌LONG-SIGHT

In long-sight, also called far-sight or technically hypermetropia, vision is usually better for distant objects than for reading. The eye is too short. Long-sight is present in most infants at birth to the extent of two or three dioptres, gradually decreasing as the eye grows. About half the population remain long-sighted to some degree during adulthood.

Parallel light rays from a distant object are not converged sufficiently, being intercepted by the retina before coming to a focus, producing a blurred image.

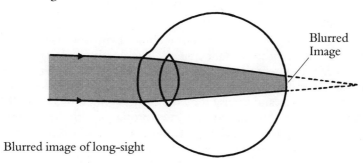

Blurred
Image

Blurred image of long-sight

If the long-sight is not too great a healthy youngster unconsciously obtains clear distance vision by accommodating to focus the light rays on the macula. However, in a young adult this constant effort by the ciliary muscle may cause visual fatigue, especially towards the end of the working day, and is dependent on the amount of long-sight.

Moreover, the additional accommodative effort required for near vision causes eye pain after long use, blurring of the image, sleepiness while reading, frontal headache, and smarting and watering of the eye. In children this may cause them to become disinterested in reading and may cause one or both eyes to turn inwards, resulting in a squint where the eyes appear crossed. Before spectacles relieved these symptoms, giving up work and long sea-voyages were considered appropriate treatment.

The sufferer must be fitted with a convex lens to converge the light rays from the distant object before they enter the eye, so that the light rays are focused on the macula without the eye accommodating.

The power of the convex lens necessary to move the focus backward onto the macula is a measure of the amount of long-sightedness. The degree of long-sightedness may be classified as low (up to three dioptres), medium (three to five dioptres) and high thereafter.

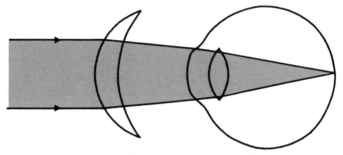

Convex lens correcting long-sight

▮ SHORT-SIGHT

In short-sight, also called near-sight or technically myopia, vision is clear for reading but fuzzy for distant objects. The eye is too long and may appear more prominent than normal. Short-sight is rare at birth, usually developing after the fourth year of life. Short-sight tends to increase during the late teens and levels off by the early twenties. In a minority of cases the eye may continue to elongate throughout life 'degenerative short-sight' leading to a retinal degeneration or even detachment,. In old age there is a tendency to increasing short-sight from cataract. Short-sight is unique to mankind affecting about thirty percent of the population, being more prevalent amongst those who engage in abundant close work. Some authorities *controversially* believe that sustained reading at too close a distance in a poor light, requires an unnatural amount of accommodation and influences the rate of progression of short-sight.

Parallel light rays from a distant object are converged to focus in front of the retina, and after crossing, continue on to form a blurred image on the retina.

A young individual cannot overcome short-sight by accommodating as this blurs distance vision even more. Since short-sight develops gradually the individual may not be aware of the deteriorating distance vision and

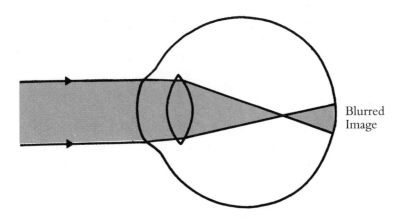

Blurred
Image

Blurred image of short-sight

may try unconsciously to improve vision by frowning, as this squeezes the lids together creating the effect of a pinhole, but this may cause fatigue headaches and lid irritation, often interpreted as light sensitivity. In dim light the pupils dilate which makes vision relatively worse.

Short-sight is corrected by concave lenses to diverge the light rays from the distant object before they enter the eye, so that the light rays are focused on the macula.

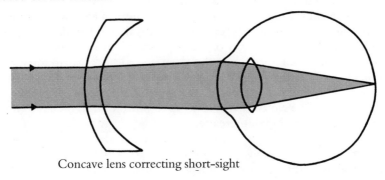

Concave lens correcting short-sight

The power of the concave lens necessary to move the focus forward onto the macula is a measure of the amount of short-sightedness. The degree of short-sightedness may be classified as low (up to three dioptres), medium (three to six dioptres), high (six to ten dioptres) and very high thereafter. Spectacles or contact lenses should not be regarded as a crutch which will be habit-forming, but used freely to enjoy comfortable and clear distance vision. People with a high degree of short-sightedness should avoid violent sports such as boxing, rugby, high diving and bungee jumping, which frequently involve trauma to the eye, as they have an increased risk of retinal detachment.

As an object approaches a naked short-sighted eye there is a finite point, dependent on the amount of the short-sightedness, where the object is seen clearly by inhibiting the accommodative effort. For example, a short-sighted person of magnitude three dioptres will be able to read at the convenient reading distance of thirty-three centimetres effortlessly without spectacles.

▌ ASTIGMATISM

Astigmatism ('not at a point'), may change in amount during life, causing indistinct, distorted vision for both distant objects and reading. In the long-sighted and short-sighted eye the curvature of the cornea is equal in all directions being spherical like a soccer ball. In the astigmatic eye the curvature of the cornea is not equal in all directions, usually the vertical meridian is steeper than the horizontal meridian, being elliptical like a rugby ball.

Light rays from an object are not converged equally in both meridians and so do not focus at a common point. Instead, vertical light rays are converged more acutely than horizontal light rays, so that two focal lines are formed at different distances from the retina

Astigmatism is corrected by a concave cylindrical lens, which operates on the light rays entering the eye in the vertical meridian only, to restore a spherical effect. The power of the concave cylindrical lens necessary to move the focal line formed by the steeper vertical meridian forward, to coincide with the focal line formed by the horizontal meridian, to create a focal point, is a measure of the amount of astigmatism. The degree of astigmatism may be classified as low (up to one dioptre), medium (one to three dioptres), and high thereafter.

Those with low astigmatism may almost constantly try to achieve a clearer, though distorted image by rapidly changing focus between the two focal lines: this may cause headaches and painful eyes, particularly for activities that require prolonged attention at a distance, such as driving. There may be a tendency to half close the lids to make a horizontal slit to cut off the light rays in the vertical meridian and obtain a more distinct image. Reading matter may be held very close to the eyes to obtain a larger, though blurred image.

In high astigmatism the image is so blurred that the effort and pain of focusing usually results in the person making no attempt to do so. However, when an adult's eyes are first corrected, circles will appear elongated into ovals until the adaptation process compensates.

Any long-sight or short-sight which is usually also present must additionally be corrected by a spherical lens. The final optical correction is a combination of a cylindrical and a spherical lens known as a toric lens, and should be worn at all times to relieve the symptoms. This was first tried in 1825 by Sir George Airy; he later became Astronomer Royal.

5.3 SUMMING-UP

The optical correction of sight defects is desirable as early in life as possible to improve vision, or to relieve eyestrain and headaches related to visual effort. However, the majority of headaches are unrelated to sight defects. Sight defects are neither induced nor prevented by wearing or not wearing spectacles or contact lenses. The eyes are not damaged by reading in poor light, sitting too close to a television, excessive use, or wearing spectacles or contact lenses with the incorrect prescription.

It should be realised that a new spectacle prescription may initially cause visual distortions and a feeling of uneasiness. During this adaptation period the visual scene may appear to slant slightly up, down or to one side. Judging distances may be disrupted as objects may appear larger, interpreted as being closer than normal, or smaller, interpreted as being farther away than normal. A minor change in prescription may be tolerated immediately or within a few hours, while a significant change may take several days of adjustment. Wearing the spectacles constantly and altering bad visual habits reduces the adaptation period.

6 | The eye examination explained

Details of previous eye injury, disease, surgery or ongoing treatment at a hospital, will be sought, including any family history of short-sight, squint, cataract, diabetes or glaucoma. Many general disorders may also affect the eye, for example, heart, artery and kidney problems, anaemia and arthritis. It is important to relate the names of any medication, potions or lotions, that are being taken as they may have side-effects; an example would be chloroquine taken for malaria which may cause blurriness when reading.

Relate when the current problem began, under what conditions, its rate of development and what action has been taken to rectify it. A full and frank account may safely be related as the information will be treated in strict confidence. The investigation and treatment will be directed to relieving the main complaint without introducing new difficulties.

Central vision in each eye is determined by noting the smallest size of letters which can be read correctly on a chart. The chart was devised in 1862 by the Dutch ophthalmologist Herman Snellen and consists of a series of high contrast letters of varying size. Each line of letters are just distinguishable by the average person when viewed at their marked distances of five, six, nine, twelve, eighteen, twenty-four, thirty-six and sixty metres.

The chart is usually viewed at six metres, so the average person is able to read down to the six metre line of letters, this is expressed as 6/6. Those only managing to read down to the twelve metre line of letters have below average vision, expressed as 6/12; they see at six metres what the average person could see at twelve metres. Those able to read even the five metre line of letters have above average vision, expressed as 6/5; they see at six metres what the average person could only see at five metres. In North America the testing distance is twenty feet; hence, average vision is expressed as 20/20. For illiterates and pre-school children vision is usually assessed with pictures or symbols.

To detect the presence of a squint or eyeturn, each eye is briefly

A
60

G W
36

O S B
24

N K H A
18

P V N U E
12

D P A S W K
9

T D E H V Y N
6

L W I R G H B O
5

covered then uncovered alternately, while staring fixedly at a letter either on the Snellen chart or at the reading distance. The optometrist carefully gauges the direction (in, out, up or down) and amount of any eye movement.

To assess the ability to move both eyes in unison, the patient reports any double vision while tracking a small object, moved close to the face in the sign of the cross. Any anomaly must be investigated to help regain the ability to use both eyes together normally to enjoy comfortable, binocular vision.

Hereditary colour vision defects are transmitted through the female, occurring in about 8% of males and 0.4% of females, the majority being of the red-green variety. This restricts careers in the armed services and merchant navy, civil aviation, police and fire services, train drivers and electricians. Colour vision defects acquired in later life are usually found in only one eye and are an early indication of disorders of the retina or optic nerve. The most popular screening test for colour vision deficiency is the Ishihara book of plates, first published in 1917. Each plate consists of a number of small dots of red and green of varying sizes, shades and intensities. One colour of dots is arranged as a number against a background of dots of the other colour. Those with normal colour vision see the number stand out. The person with defective colour vision confuses the camouflaged number and sees either another number or no definite pattern.

An uncomfortable trial frame containing blurring lenses will be fitted and the lights dimmed creating a very relaxing atmosphere. Whilst looking straight ahead the temptation to close the eyes should be resisted, although blinking is permitted. Using a hand-held retinoscope, a torch with a mirror on top, the optometrist shines a light into the eye. By exchanging lenses in the trial frame, dependent on the movement of the light reflected from the retina, it is possible to gauge reasonably accurately the prescription. It will also indicate a corneal defect, cataract or dirty soft contact lens. When the lights come up the results obtained provide a starting point for a refining procedure.

There are two methods for determining astigmatism, they are of equal value although some people respond better to one test than to the other.

The older method requires the viewing of radial lines spread out in a semicircle at regular intervals, resembling a fan.

By identifying the orientation of the clearest radial line, the appropriate cylindrical lens is introduced to render all the radial lines equally clear. This test has more scope to be misunderstood than any other. Check

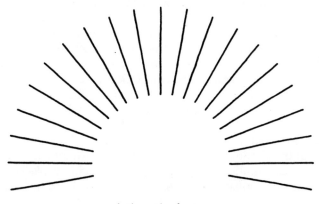

Astigmatic chart

yourself by looking at the above dial at arm's length, one eye at a time with and without spectacles.

The newer method, first used a century ago, requires rotating a special lens, mounted on a handle, held before the eye. While viewing a small target two choices are presented in quick succession. By making a slight adjustment to the cylindrical lens, performing a twirl and making a fresh appeal, the astigmatic component is eventually revealed when the choices appear equal.

To balance the spherical component of the eyes, attention is directed to two black rings, one on a red background and the other on a green background. One ring usually appears blacker, clearer and sharper, by changing the trial lenses the rings are made to appear equal. Some may get thoroughly confused by this test, but it is important not to guess. This test is equally valid for colour vision defectives.

Near vision is assessed by the ability to read varying sizes of 'Times New Roman' type print, measured by the printers' point system, one point being one seventy-second of an inch. Normal near vision is expressed as N5, which is attainable for those with 6/12 or better on the Snellen chart. If text of this size cannot be read or only with a struggle then the additional lens power necessary to restore comfortable reading at the desired position must be determined. The size of the average newspaper column is N8.

When visiting the optician it is essential to take both outdoor and reading spectacles, to judge if the improvement seems significant. Lenses should be cleaned beforehand as sometimes impairment of vision is little more than grossly restricted light transmission. Frequent changes in the prescription could be an indication of uncontrolled diabetes.

The interior of the eye is examined for health using a hand-held ophthalmoscope, a torch with a mirror and lenses, which gives a view of the lens, vitreous and retina, with a magnification of fifteen. A bright light is directed into the eye from very close proximity for a couple of minutes. This creates a temporary coloured after-image which may last a few minutes.

Those interested in contact lens wear have the front of the eye scrutinised by a double-barrelled microscope mounted horizontally, which gives a magnification of up to fifty. The chin is placed on a rest, while a lamp on a movable mechanical arm shines a dazzling beam of light accurately on to the eye.

There are two different methods for measuring the eye pressure to detect or monitor chronic glaucoma, which affects about half a percent of adults over the age of forty years.

The most accurate method, common amongst ophthalmologists, is to apply a small probe illuminated with a blue light gently onto the anaesthetised cornea. However, the instillation of anaesthetic drops initially causes stinging, similar to having soap in the eye.

A painless though less precise method, popular with optometrists, requires a sudden, explosive puff of air to be directed on to the eye, flattening the cornea. Since it takes less time to flatten a soft eye than a hard eye, the time taken relates to the eye pressure.

A more sensitive test for establishing the presence and effect of chronic glaucoma is to chart any typical visual field loss within the total area of vision of each eye. There are various ways of doing this, the most common technique employed by optometrists is to flash in quick succession various patterns of dots of light, which are made gradually brighter, until they are just observed.

7 | Choosing type of correction

There are various elective surgical operations designed to overcome sight defects, although spectacles or contact lenses will almost always additionally be required to attain optimal distance vision, which in a few cases will be permanently poorer than that previously enjoyed. This treatment is not suitable for children, as their eyes are still growing making re-correction necessary. Naturally, the advisability of any intended treatment should be discussed with the general practitioner (GP).

Approximately five percent of people in Britain wear contact lenses, although with rare exceptions they are intended to complement spectacles rather than being a full-time replacement.

7.1 SURGICAL CORRECTION

Healthy adults with stable short-sight, in the range from two to ten dioptres, may choose from two surgical procedures to enable clearer distance vision without spectacles or contact lenses. However, reading spectacles will then be required by the middle aged. Radial keratotomy (RK) and photorefractive keratectomy (PRK) both correct short-sight by making fine alterations to the shape of the cornea, so that images are focused more accurately on the macula. The main problem is the lack of predictability of the final outcome, especially for high short-sightedness, as the body's healing process is variable. Any residual optical correction required by fitting contact lenses is more problematic in RK than PRK, since the shape of the cornea bulges forward.

Laser thermo keratoplasty (LTK) is an *experimental* procedure for the surgical correction of up to five dioptres of long-sightedness using the infrared holmium laser. A strict protocol requires that patients must be over twenty-one years old, and have stable vision.

■ RADIAL KERATOTOMY (RK)

Radial keratotomy, the so-called 'Russian Operation' which Dr Fyodorov refined in the 1970's, is popular in the US and has been available in Britain since the early 1980's. Using a micrometer-set

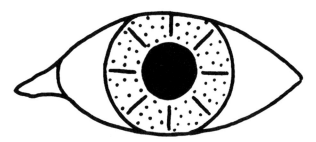

Radial incisions

diamond knife up to sixteen radial incisions are made in the peripheral cornea, thereby avoiding the central optical zone through which the eye sees. The number, length and direction of the incisions are dependent on the corneal thickness and the amount of short-sightedness. The cornea is maintained in its curvature by the intraocular eye pressure and the elasticity of its own tissues. Generally eight incisions weaken the cornea sufficiently to allow a controlled amount of expansion to create a flatter cornea, thereby reducing the short-sight.

The operation takes a few minutes and is carried out under anaesthesia. Mild postoperative discomfort is commonly felt for twenty-four to forty-eight hours. The second eye is operated on after several weeks. Any increased flexibility in the eyeball may cause daily fluctuations in sharpness of vision; this usually settles after a month or two. The need for incisions up to ninety-five percent of the corneal thickness, causes permanent scarring, which may never totally heal, with an increased risk of rupture if the eye should suffer blunt trauma. Light may be scattered by these scars in a sunburst pattern and cause unusual sensitivity to bright light. Glare is typically worse at night when the pupil is dilated. Corneal ulcers have been reported and inadvertent corneal perforation has led to cataract and infection within the eye.

In about one in four progressive changes occur up to five years after surgery, this leads to long-sightedness which may be distressing. It is now standard procedure to aim to leave the patient slightly short-sighted to allow for this change. Patients with less than five dioptres of short-sightedness preoperatively achieve 6/6 in fifty percent of cases, while those of a higher degree preoperatively fare worse, especially the under thirty-five year olds.

▌PHOTOREFRACTIVE KERATECTOMY (PRK)

Photorefractive keratectomy, first investigated in 1983, has been available in Britain since 1989. Re-profiling of the cornea is achieved with an excimer laser, which produces a narrow, uniform beam of invisible ultraviolet light energy, but no heat. This energy is used to break down molecular bonds and vaporise corneal tissue with only a minimal adverse effect on immediately adjacent corneal tissue.

Anaesthetic drops are instilled into the eye and the surface cells of the cornea in the central optical zone are mechanically scraped away, this takes several minutes. Then while the patient stares at a fixed light, the laser ablates the cornea, by successive pulses lasting only seconds, heard as a tapping sound. A computer connected to the laser controls the progressive opening of a diaphragm, which regulates the amount of tissue removed from the central cornea, based on the reduction in short-sightedness desired. Typically about ten percent of corneal thickness is removed, creating a flatter cornea. The patient is able to return home within the hour, but strong pain killers are issued for the severe postoperative pain, particularly at night, this can last for three to five days.

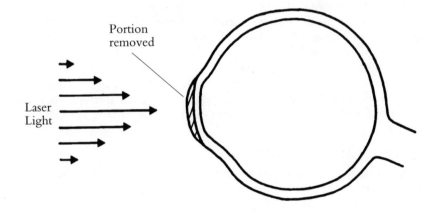

Photorefractive keratectomy (PRK)

The remodelled cornea heals in the ensuing weeks, during which the eye will not see properly. The second eye would not be treated for at least three months, often six months, to allow the first eye to stabilise and the result to be assessed. During this period binocular vision may be attainable by wearing a contact lens in the unoperated eye.

The results of treatment may not be permanent and any complications or side effects may require additional treatment. The more the amount of short-sightedness corrected, so the greater the variability of the result. Patients with less than six dioptres of short-sightedness preoperatively achieve the driving test standard in eighty-five percent of cases, but in patients with more than six dioptres the predictability of the results are significantly less, with a tendency for regression towards pre-surgical status. To reverse regression and reduce troublesome central corneal haze, which causes glare especially noticeable at night, steroid eye drops are given for three months, but this may have the side effect of raising the intraocular eye pressure.

Long-term results and possible complications are unknown. Complaints recorded, which may be temporary or permanent, include persistent foreign body sensation, tenderness on rubbing the eye, infection and delayed corneal healing. At night when the pupils dilate, if the transition zone between the central treated area of the cornea and the untreated area beyond is visible, a disabling halo effect is experienced.

▮ LASER THERMO KERATOPLASTY (LTK)

Eight points in the tissue of the cornea, forming a circle around the pupil, each receive a three-second burst of infrared laser beam focused as a mini cone of intense heat. The widest part of the cone is at the outer surface of the cornea, so that the shrinking tissue will create a steeper cornea, reducing the long-sight. For severe long-sight a further eight points, in a second wider circle, are targetted. Sight is usually normal after a week but the laser points remain as small marks on the surface of the eye for up to a year.

7.2 OPTICAL CORRECTION

Contact lenses involve a commitment of time and money, and should not be entered into without some thought to the practical considerations and potential hazards, compared to spectacles.

▮ COSMETIC

Spectacles have a high profile and can be considered as facial adornment. Sympathetically chosen spectacles may flatter the appearance, but when removed leave unsightly little red pressure marks, where supported on the nose and ears. With higher power spectacle lenses especially, the eye will appear smaller for a short-sighted person and larger for a long-sighted person.

Contact lenses will only be visible if that is the intention, for example to change the apparent colour of the eye.

■ CONVENIENCE

Spectacles may be worn for any duration and whenever the need arises, without preparation.

Contact lenses require adherence to a wearing schedule. The wearing time is increased each day to allow the eyes to adapt gradually to the contact lens. Contact lenses cannot be inserted or removed with the same speed or casualness as spectacles. Clean hands and fingernails, trimmed short, are prerequisites for handling the contact lenses in the daily time-consuming ritual of keeping them clean. Those whose hands are regularly ingrained with dirt, oil or grease, are not suitable. The adjustment period in learning to use contact lenses properly is longer than with spectacles.

■ OPTICAL

Spectacle wearers have their *clear* field of view restricted by the size of the spectacle lens, and become accustomed to the presence of the spectacle frame in their peripheral field of view.

Contact lenses move with the eye so wearers have no restriction of their field of view.

Spectacle lenses can give annoying reflections, especially visible at night. People with short-sightedness of more than four dioptres are handicapped by the small image size produced by the spectacle lens. People who have had a cataract removed, without having an intraocular lens replacement, suffer from the large image size produced by the spectacle lens.

Contact lenses offer the advantage of a more normal image size by being closer to the eye, and eliminate the aberrations and peripheral distortions of the thick spectacle lens, giving better vision.

■ SAFETY

Spectacles glazed with shatterproof lenses afford some measure of protection from flying objects by virtue of their physical presence deflecting the oncoming projectile. However, professional athletes can participate in competitive sports only by being free of the encumbrance and hazard of spectacles.

In the event of a chemical splash to the eye, the chemical agent may seep beneath the contact lens to cause extensive damage before the contact lens can be removed.

Contact lenses poorly fitted, improperly inserted or removed, or with an insufficient tear circulation, can cause corneal abrasions and ulcers. Wearers should be able to distinguish between symptoms that can be expected and tolerated, from those that are danger signals requiring contact lens removal or indicating immediate consultation, for example persistent red eyes, blurring of vision, excessive glare, disproportionate watering or unusual discomfort. The maxim to follow is "If in doubt, have them out", which should be engraved on all contact lens cases.

■ ENVIRONMENT

Rain and perspiration deposit on spectacle lenses and steam up when the wearer goes from the cold outside into a warm room. Spectacles are not compatible with using certain types of optical aids, for example binoculars, and with wearing some protective helmets or masks.

The hot, dry, dusty, smoky atmospheres encountered in office buildings, or the very windy conditions experienced in a speeding convertible car, will not affect spectacle wearers, but may be an inconvenience to contact lens wearers.

Contact lenses are contraindicated where there is: a likelihood of injury from industrial hazards, for example welders' flash burns ('arc eye'), intense heat or cold; in a highly particulate, acidic or alkali atmosphere; low humidity; at high altitude.

■ MEDICAL

Contact lenses are recommended to mask a disfiguring feature, for example an absence or irregularity of the iris, to flatten a bulging cone-shaped deformed cornea, to protect the cornea from turned-in eyelashes, to relieve the pain of a blistered cornea and to promote healing of an injured cornea.

Where small corneal scars create an irregular corneal surface, vision is greatly improved by the smooth surface of a contact lens.

Contact lenses are contraindicated in allergic and inflammatory conditions, for example hay fever, when there is an abnormal over or under production of tears, when the eyelids are lax, in a protruding eye or in the presence of a marked pterygium.

Contact lens wearers need to have regular eye check-ups.

■ FINANCIAL

Spectacles are virtually maintenance-free, whereas contact lenses require costly solutions for on-going daily aftercare.

8 | Contact lenses

Leonardo da Vinci conceived and sketched prototype contact lenses in 1508. Contact lenses are finely fashioned, thin discs, about the size of a fingernail, that correct most sight defects for which spectacles, including bifocals, would normally be worn.

Practical glass contact lenses, moistened with a sterilised solution of grape sugar, were tried in the early twentieth century, but they were not to everybody's taste as they could only be tolerated for about two hours, due to the excessive weight.

In 1938, a plastic material called polymethyl methacrylate (PMMA) replaced glass as it was lighter, shatter-proof and easily moulded. Developments in the early 1980's combined silicone and fluorocarbon with PMMA to create gas-permeable **rigid contact lenses**.

In 1965, a new plastic polymer material hydroxyethyl methacrylate (HEMA) was patented which absorbs water to become soft and pliable. Since then, new polymers have been added to produce **soft contact lenses**.

All contact lenses need rigorous hygiene in their daily routine aftercare, with various special solutions and tablets, to avoid spoiling by con-

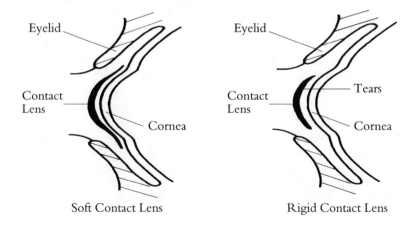

Soft Contact Lens   Rigid Contact Lens

tamination and to minimise the risk of irritation or infection of the eye. The contact lens case should be replaced frequently and cleaned weekly to remove germs.

However, even an optimally fitted contact lens is a foreign body, with an element of risk of acute or long-term eye damage dependent on the length of time worn. There is a very low incidence of contact lens induced microbial corneal inflammation; the risk is least with daily wear gas–permeable rigid contact lenses, and greatest with soft contact lenses worn overnight.

8.1 RIGID CONTACT LENSES

A rigid contact lens floats on a continuous tear cushion over the cornea, the 'surface tension' making it adhere quite strongly. By matching the contour of the back surface of the rigid contact lens to the exact measurement of the curvature of the cornea, the pressure of the contact lens is evenly distributed over the cornea. The profile of the front surface of a rigid contact lens determines the power, dictated by the wearer's prescription.

The edge of a rigid contact lens is thin, rounded and polished, so that it can gently slide underneath the upper eyelid during blinking without being dislodged. Blinking properly is important, to maintain a tear film on the front surface of the rigid contact lens, and to pump tears under the contact lens to supply the cornea with oxygen. The thinner the central thickness of the rigid contact lens, the more comfortable and greater the oxygen transmission, but the less stable, and more likely the contact lens is to warp and break.

To allow the eye to tolerate the presence of a rigid contact lens the length of time it is worn is gradually increased every day, over a few weeks, until the desired maximum daily wearing time is achieved. During this adaptation period, there is an awareness of the rigid contact lens in the eye, excessive blinking, watering of the eyes, light sensitivity and temporary blurred vision when switching directly back to spectacles. When resuming wear after a few days abstinence tolerance will need to be restored by progressively increasing the wearing time as before.

PMMA hard contact lenses are extremely stable and biocompatible, but are impermeable to oxygen such that long–term wearers may experience a reduced corneal sensitivity, severe spectacle blur after lens removal and abnormal corneas. They have been superseded by gas-permeable rigid contact lenses which have a greater oxygen and carbon dioxide permeability. These are more flexible while retaining the ability to correct moderate amounts of astigmatism and wet more easily to permit better tear flow beneath them. They are made of cellulose acetate butyrate (CAB), silicone, fluorocarbon, or combinations, and have a life expectancy of up to five years.

The advantages of silicone-based combinations are easier and faster adaptation, greater comfort and increased wearing time. Their large size gives better vision and reduced glare from lights at night, despite the healthy movement of the lens with blinking. The improved thermal conductivity of the material permits greater heat dissipation, through the contact lens, reducing the corneal oxygen demand. The drawbacks are fragility, with a tendency to chip or scratch, and more susceptibility to deposits, requiring regular cleaning, which adds to the maintenance.

Fluorocarbon is similar to Teflon used in non-stick frying pans and gives rigid contact lenses lighter weight, deposit resistance and greatly increased oxygen permeability, giving potential for extended wear.

It is essential that the wearer is fully instructed on how to insert, remove, re-centre and care for their rigid contact lenses, and to recognise symptoms that could result in serious corneal damage. Severe pain can result from grit getting under a rigid contact lens, but do not rub the eye with the contact lens in place. A poorly fitted rigid contact lens may also scratch, abrade or erode the cornea. This could produce a painful red eye that obscures vision and provides an entry point for bacteria to form an ulcer. Body-contact sports such as football should be avoided as there is a risk of dislodgement. Swimming should also be avoided as the lenses are easily washed out.

Before inserting a rigid contact lens, a wetting solution is applied so that the tear film spreads easily and evenly on both surfaces of the contact lens, ensuring comfort and good vision. It is important to insert rigid contact lenses before any cosmetic is applied to the eyelids, and to avoid oil-based cosmetics altogether. When a rigid contact lens is removed from the eye it will be covered with mucus, crystalline deposits, and oily and sebaceous secretions. These materials must be removed daily by applying a suitable cleaner before storage. Soaking solutions used overnight also clean the rigid contact lens; they contain germicidal agents to disinfect the contact lens and keep it hydrated.

8.2 SOFT CONTACT LENSES

The hydrophilic soft contact lens has the ability to absorb water to become highly elastic and soft, yet remaining strong, while holding its shape and dimensions. However, if it is allowed to dry out it becomes distorted, hard and brittle, being easily broken. The higher the water content of the soft contact lens, the greater the oxygen transmission to the cornea, but the less durable and the more fragile it becomes. The thinner the soft contact lens, the greater the oxygen transmission to the cornea, although it will tear more easily and wrinkling may reduce vision. A soft contact lens slightly touches the centre and periphery of the eye.

Soft contact lenses are suitable for extended wear, if they are very thin or have over seventy percent water content, but require careful monitoring by the fitter. With long-term wear, mineral, protein and fat deposits may accumulate on the surface; these reduce vision, reduce oxygen transmission, and may cause swelling of the conjunctiva lining the eyelid and a red eye.

The advantages of soft contact lenses are immediate exceptional comfort and lack of awareness during normal blinking, since there is almost no interference to the upper eyelids from the thin edges of the lens. Tolerance is extremely rapid, this allows intermittent wear so that they may be worn for several hours on special occasions. They are ideal for any kind of vigorous physical activity, especially sports, as accidental dislodgement is unlikely. When switching directly back to spectacles there is no temporary blur to vision as experienced with rigid contact lenses. There is no glare or light sensitivity which is seen in the early weeks of rigid contact lens wear.

A disadvantage of soft contact lenses is that not much astigmatism is corrected, as the soft contact lens contours itself to the misshapen cornea, giving poor or variable vision. Soft contact lenses are much more fragile than rigid contact lenses, having a life expectancy of up to eighteen months. They are prone to tearing, especially during insertion and removal. The adherence to a cleaning and disinfection procedure is most important, even if the soft contact lenses are unused for a period, or infection may occur.

Soft contact lenses should not be worn in the presence of irritating fumes, vapour or hair spray. If vision is blurred while wearing soft contact lenses the contact lens may be inside out, off centre, not clean, or right and left contact lenses may have been accidentally switched. The soft contact lens should be removed for inspection, cleaned, rinsed and reinserted. Do not use tap water, particularly if it comes from a storage tank, distilled water or spring water, as a substitute for saline for use with soft contact lenses. Tears naturally contain many types of protein which gradually build up on the soft contact lens despite daily cleaning. A weekly enzyme cleaner is necessary to break down the protein deposits.

'Disposable' soft contact lenses are discarded and replaced with a new pair daily, weekly or fortnightly, while frequent replacement programmes supply fresh lenses at regular intervals of between one to six months. Wearers whose contact lenses are frequently spoiled by the build up of deposits, prolonged wear, rough handling or poor adherence to the strict care regime, are better suited to this mode of wear.

Transparent tinted soft contact lenses will enhance or darken the colour of the eyes, but for dramatic eye colour changes, solid tinted soft contact lenses are necessary to mask the underlying colour, although the appearance is less natural.

9 | Frames

When the famous Venetian merchant Marco Polo served the court of Kublai Khan in China in 1270, he initially mistook courtiers, wearing ready-made reading spectacles, for jesters. Demand picked up in the late fifteenth century when printed books became available, but it was not until the seventeenth century that elaborately-worked frames of gold, silver or tortoiseshell were commonly employed by the fashionable set.

Pince-nez are now passé; the ease with which they can be brought into use and removed is offset by their strong grip on the nose which alters the nasal tone. Monocles, now outdated are rarely favoured. Semi-rimless frames have the lens retained by a thin nylon cord hidden in a groove, usually around the lower edge. Rimless frames have no apparent material holding the lens shape.

2.1 FRAME MATERIALS

Metal frames are made of gold, silver, nickel, stainless steel, anodised aluminium, titanium and alloys. They usually have two adjustable plastic pads, useful to accurately place bifocal lenses before the eye, while pure silicon soft pads also prevent slipping and pressure marks.

There are two methods for the production of plastic frames, a low-quality injection-moulding and a higher-quality cutting from a sheet. Cellulose nitrate is not used now as it burns fiercely if ignited, and becomes brittle and yellow with age. Nylon is injection-moulded becoming brittle with age. Cellulose acetate is in most common use being available in various colours and patterns. Perspex is tougher and retains its shape requiring more heat for manipulation. Carbon fibre is lightweight and tougher but expensive. Optyl is thirty percent lighter than cellulose acetate, more fire-resistant, biologically inert and returns to its original position after distortion by undue tension. A plastic frame keeps its adjustment well once fitted and, usually, has a fixed nosepiece.

Tortoiseshell from the hawksbill turtle is now extremely rare. Solid is preferable to spliced, with blonde or demi-blonde being more expensive. Fish-bone, horn, wood and leather have been used but have now been superseded by other materials.

2.2 FRAME SELECTION

The face is the first feature noticed and assessed when forming a first impression, the eyes being the greatest source of expression reflecting the personality. A suitably chosen frame complementing hair and eye colour, skin tone and face shape, enhances the appearance without drawing attention to itself. The shape of the frame (round, oval, heart, rectangular or square) should not match the face shape. Frames should meet these essentials:

- Frames for distance should sit vertically, whereas frames for reading should be slightly lowered and tilted downward.
- The nasal side of the frame, or lens in the case of rimless, must conform to the contour of the side of the nose.
- For regular-sized spectacles, it is preferable for the upper rim to leave at least part of the eyebrow visible above it.
- The frame should not be so deep that it rests on the cheeks, as it will be uncomfortable and may become discoloured by make-up and perspiration. A shallow frame is essential for plump cheeks.
- The frame should not irritate the skin where it is supported on the ears and nose. Some people are allergic to certain types of metal frames, especially in humid tropical conditions.

A large nose is in good company with a large, thick frame with a saddle nosepiece. A long nose can be concealed by positioning the bridge so that its line cuts across the nose as low as possible, the effect being accentuated by dark colours. A petite nose may be emphasised by a slender bridge set high or a keyhole bridge, to add nasal length giving more balance to the face. Dark coloured frames draw attention to nose width and should be avoided by people with very narrow or very wide noses.

For close-set eyes, a wide frame will make the appearance worse. Close-set eyes can be made to look wider apart by choosing a frame with a clear bridge area graduating to a deeper colour at the outer edge or frames that are greater in depth at the outer ends than at the middle.

Long faces can be 'shortened' by frames with low set joints which are noticeably longer horizontally than vertically. Shallow faces can be 'lengthened' by frames with high set joints. Avoid choosing a larger than necessary frame, for momentarily fashionable considerations, as it will add to the weight and be cosmetically challenging especially with high power lenses.

Select colour with care, for instance blue can look cold and red warm. The eye's own colour will be heightened by a frame of a contrasting colour, for example, when blue and green are juxtaposed, the blue looks bluer and the green looks greener. Gold is most attractive on dark skin, bright colours favour olive skin, while light colours are better for fair complexions.

For most people one frame is not suitable for every occasion. Several frames may be necessary to adequately encompass an individual's various activities. Those relying on spectacles for a particular use, for example driving, should always keep spare spectacles in case of loss or breakage. Prescription sunglasses are useful and practical, especially for outgoing people. If the spectacles are to be worn constantly, comfort is the overriding factor. If for active sports safety and security are paramount, and if they are to be taken on and off frequently, stoutness is most important.

9.3 SAFETY SPECTACLES

All safety spectacles conforming and tested to British Standard, BS 2092, have a kitemark on both frame and lenses according to the grade. Safety spectacles offer primary protection against optical radiation and impact from flying particles, although without a side shield only frontal protection is afforded. When greater protection is demanded, for example when working with chemicals, welding or lathes, professional guidance on suitable goggles, face shield or helmet must be sought.

Ball games and racket sports can be dangerous, especially squash, since the ball is small enough to fit inside the protective bony rim of the eye socket to cause a very serious eye injury. In the event of an accident medical attention should be sought as soon as possible. Goggles make working outdoors under a car safer from wind blowing dust or rust into the eyes.

Sun lamp users, arc welders subject to 'arc eye' and skiers vulnerable to 'snow-blindness', must wear protective filters to guard against invisible ultraviolet radiation damaging the cornea. Otherwise several hours later **both** eyes will be uniformly red over the exposed area, feel gritty, accompanied in severe cases by dislike of bright light and intense pain, which may be relieved by the application of an ice pack or cold water. Patching the eyes for twenty-four hours allows the cornea to heal completely.

Photographers handling developers and fixers should take care not to rub their eyes. Should chemicals get on to the eye, separate the eyelids immediately and flood the eye with cool water for at least ten minutes and, if possible, open the eyes under water. Alkali burns are more serious and penetrating than acid burns, and both require further medical assessment.

The eyes require protection for DIY grinding, electric sanding, chipping, hammering, chiselling or drilling, as small particles of metal, glass or brick, can fly off at high speed and become embedded in the cornea or even enter the eye. Corneal foreign bodies cause pain, light sensitivity and copious watering. By shining a torch obliquely the particle is seen as a dark opacity, which in the case of a metal is surrounded by a stained rust ring after six to eight hours. Do not try to remove an embedded particle, cover the eye with a pad and seek medical care as soon as possible. After removal healing is usually complete within twenty-four hours, but may take as long as four days and leave a scar. Strangely the more serious penetrating eye injury, requiring emergency surgery, may not be felt on penetration and leave no visible entry wound.

10 | VDUs

The Health and Safety (Display Screen Equipment) Regulations 1992, requires employers to provide VDU and microfiche users with an eye examination at regular intervals and to reduce associated health risks, such as repetitive strain injury, upper limb disorders, visual fatigue and mental stress. Employers have a responsibility to provide suitable spectacles only if they are required solely for VDU use, which is likely to apply to 5-10% of employees; for example, VDU users who normally wear spectacles or contact lenses for reading, where the screen or the documents are positioned beyond their usual reading distance, or where the height of the screen would require bifocal wearers to adopt an unnatural head posture, to allow viewing through the reading segment, causing neck or back aches.

To efficiently use a VDU for a prolonged period on a daily basis without visual fatigue requires that the operator must have optimum vision, suitable lighting, equipment in good adjustment and takes frequent short breaks to relax the eyes by looking into the far distance. A few users find tinted, polarising or anti-reflection coated lenses beneficial. A document holder attached to the left of the screen significantly reduces fatigue from excessive movements of the eyes and neck.

Users with an uncorrected sight defect or poor eye co-ordination, lacking the high standard of vision necessary to successfully cope with the visually demanding nature of VDU work, may experience for the first time some of the following symptoms, given in order of reported frequency: eyestrain, headaches, blurred vision, light sensitivity, or double vision.

An eye examination to correct the previously unsuspected visual deficiency may completely eliminate all symptoms. Although, it is existing spectacle wearers who complain more frequently of visually related discomfort, particularly the over forties, and those whose work is monotonous.

The concentration of VDU work is associated with a reduced blink rate, and when combined with the hot, arid atmosphere of a centrally heated office, may result in dry irritated eyes, especially for contact lens wearers. A colourful solution is to have fresh flowers in a vase to increase the humidity; also blinking more often and using artificial tear drops will help, and wearing spectacles in place of contact lenses for VDU work.

10.1 HOW TO IDEALLY ADJUST THE WORKSTATION
Sitting comfortably? Below, is shown the ideal body posture with corresponding height configuration of the workstation.

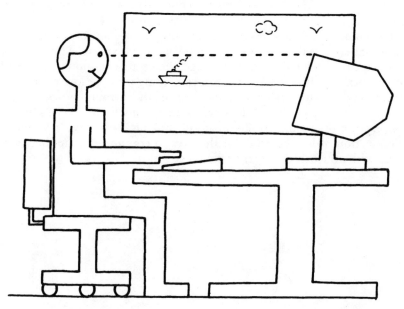

The chair should be adjusted so that the lower arms and desk are approximately parallel, this enables good keyboard technique. An upright sitting position, fully utilising the seat area, allows the properly adjusted backrest to support the lumbar region. A curved back creates one-sided stress to be placed on the spinal discs causing excessive edge wear. If feet are not firmly on the floor use a foot rest to avoid excess pressure on the backs of the lower legs and knees. To lessen stiffness, neck and backpain, which result from maintaining the same static seated position for long periods, occasional movement is recommended.

The eyes should be at the same level as the top of the VDU casing and at least an outstretched arms length distance. Angle the screen to eliminate reflections, which reduce the visibility and create focusing difficulties;

both of these cause fatigue. If there is no screen position that avoids annoying reflections from immovable light sources they should be replaced by purpose-designed lamps. Fluorescent fittings should be sited with their length at right angles to the screen face and not parallel to it. Ideally, windows should be at right angles to the screen. Since windows in front give direct glare to the operator while those behind cause reflections in the screen, they should be fitted with curtains or blinds. Occasionally, clean the screen to remove dirt, grime and finger marks. Surprisingly, fitting a screen filter to reduce glare and enhance contrast, can improve on the manufacturers' specifications.

For comfort, tweak the contrast and brightness controls to keep the contrast between the screen background and the text low. This will also lessen the harmless coloured after-images which are commonly perceived after working with a VDU. The office lighting must be low enough to minimise the contrast between the screen and the surroundings but bright enough for the legibility of documents. In a dimly lit office, consider an angle poise desk lamp to illuminate documents to achieve a balanced illumination; it is very tiring for the eyes to continually adapt between areas with noticeably different brightness.

11 | Continuing care

The representative professional organisations will provide further information.

The General Optical Council (GOC)
41 Harley Street, London WlN 2DJ. Tel: 0171-580 3898
The GOC was established by the Opticians Act 1958, to promote high standards of professional education and conduct, and to maintain two registers, one of optometrists and the other of dispensing opticians.

Association of Optometrists (AOP)
Bridge House, 233-234 Blackfriars Road, London SEl 8NW. Tel: 0171-261 9661
The AOP is an organisation that promotes and protects the professional interests of both optometrists and dispensing opticians, and encourages high standards of practice.

Optical Consumer Complaints Service (OCCS)
address as the Association of Optometrists
The OCCS came into being in January 1993 to provides a conciliation service to settle complaints from the public about optical services, spectacles or contact lenses provided by opticians.

The Federation of Ophthalmic and Dispensing Opticians (FODO)
113 Eastbourne Mews, London W2 6LQ. Tel: 0171-258 0240
The FODO was formed in July 1985 to assist registered opticians operate effectively for the benefit of the public.

Institute of Optometry
56-62 Newington Causeway, London SEl 6DS. Tel: 0171-407 4183
The Institute is staffed partly by volunteers serving the public in all aspects of general optometric and contact lens practice.

Eyecare Information Service (EIS)
PO Box 3597, London SEl 6DY. Tel: 0171-357 7730
The EIS was formed by the merger of the Eye Care Information Bureau and the Optical Information Council in 1993, to publicise the services available from opticians, the importance of eyecare, and technological innovations and fashions in spectacles and contact lenses.

International Glaucoma Association (IGA)
King's College Hospital, Denmark Hill, London SE5 9RS.
Tel: 0171-274 6222 Ext. 2934
Formed in 1974 the Association is happy to answer questions about glaucoma both on the telephone or by letter.

11.1 PROFESSIONAL QUALIFYING BODY FOR OPTOMETRISTS

The British College of Optometrists (BCO)
10 Knaresborough Place, London SW5 OTG. Tel: 0171-373 7765
The BCO was formed on 1st March 1980 and holds the Professional Qualifying Examination which provides entitlement to registration as an optometrist with the GOC. Optometrists must agree to abide by the Code of Ethics of the College which sets a high standard of professional conduct.

■ EDUCATIONAL INSTITUTIONS FOR OPTOMETRISTS

Aston University
Department of Vision Sciences
Aston Triangle, Birmingham B4 7ET
Tel: 0121-359 3611/5161

University of Bradford
Department of Optometry
Richmond Road
Bradford, Yorkshire BD7 1DP
Tel: 01274-384636

The City University
Department of Optometry and Visual Science
Dame Alice Owen Building
311-321 Goswell Road, London EC1V 7DD
Tel: 0171-477 8000

Glasgow Caledonian University
Department of Vision Sciences
Cowcaddens Road, Glasgow G4 OBA
Tel: 0141-331 3000 ext 3379

UMIST: University of Manchester Institute of Science and Technology
Department of Optometry and Visual Sciences
PO Box 88
Sackville Street, Manchester M60 1QD
Tel: 0161-200 3870

University of Wales College of Cardiff
Department of Optometry and Vision Sciences
PO Box 905, Redwood Building
King Edward VII Avenue, Cardiff CFl 3YJ
Tel: 01222-874852

11.2 PROFESSIONAL QUALIFYING BODY FOR DISPENSING OPTICIANS

Association of British Dispensing Opticians (ABDO)
6 Hurlingham Business Park, Sullivan Road, London SW6 3DU.
Tel: 0171-736 0088

The ABDO was founded in 1986 and adjudicates the qualifying examination which provides entitlement to registration as a dispensing optician with the GOC. The ABDO is a representative body for all sections of the optical dispensing profession.

∎ EDUCATIONAL INSTITUTIONS FOR DISPENSING OPTICIANS

The Association of British Dispensing Opticians
Address given above

Anglia Higher Education College
Department of Applied Sciences – Ophthalmic Dispensing
East Road, Cambridge CBl lPT
Tel 01223-352992

Bradford and Ilkley Community College
Ophthalmic Dispensing Section
Department of Science
Great Horton Road, Bradford BD7 lAY
Tel: 01274-753416

City and East London College
Bunhill Row, London EClY 8LQ
Tel: 0171-638 4171

Glasgow Caledonian University
Address given above

OTHER BOOKS FROM AMBERWOOD PUBLISHING ARE:

Aromatherapy – A Guide for Home Use by Christine Westwood. All you need to know about essential oils and using them. £1.99.

Aromatherapy for Stress Management by Christine Westwood. Covering the use of essential oils for everyday stress-related problems. £2.99.

Plant Medicine – A Guide for Home Use by Charlotte Mitchell MNIMH. Everything you need to know about plants that can be used in home treatments. £2.99.

Woman Medicine – Vitex Agnus Castus by Simon Mills MA, FNIMH. The wonderful story of the herb that has been used for centuries in the treatment of women's problems. £2.99.

Ancient Medicine – Ginkgo Biloba by Dr Desmond Corrigan BSc(Pharms), MA, Phd, FLS, FPSI. Poor memory, ageing and lack of concentration are among the symptoms which the medicine from this fascinating and ancient tree are said to cure. £2.99.

Herbal First Aid by Andrew Chevallier BA, MNIMH. A beautifully clear reference book of natural remedies and general first aid in the home. £2.99.

Indian Medicine – The Immune System by Desmond Corrigan BSc(Pharms), MA, Phd, FLS, FPSI. An intriguing account of the history and science of the plant called Echinacea and its power to influence the immune system. £2.99.

Aromatherapy – For Healthy Legs and Feet by Christine Westwood. A comprehensive guide to the use of essential oils for the treatment of legs and feet, including illustrated massage instructions. £2.99.

Signs & Symptoms of Vitamin Deficiency by Dr Leonard Mervyn BSc, PhD, C.Chem, FRCS. A home guide for self-diagnosis which explains and assesses Vitamin Therapy for the prevention of a wide variety of diseases and illnesses. £2.99.

Causes & Prevention of Vitamin Deficiency by Dr Leonard Mervyn BSc, PhD, C.Chem, FRCS. A home guide to the Vitamin content of foods and the depletion caused by cooking, storage and processing. It includes advice for those whose needs are increased due to lifestyle, illness etc. £2.99.